Y0-BDI-950

The Couch Potato Workout: 101 Exercises You Can Do At Home!

By Joel M. Press, MD
Illustrated by Dan Muir

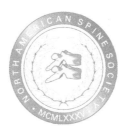

North American Spine Society
www.spine.org

© 2006, North American Spine Society
ISBN number 1-929988-15-X

The information in this book is selective and does not cover all aspects of health and exercise. If you have any questions contact your health care provider for more information. You should consult your health care provider before embarking on any exercise program. This book is for general information and understanding only and is not intended to represent official policy of the North American Spine Society. Please consult your health care provider for specific information about your condition.

North American Spine Society
22 Calendar Ct., 2nd floor
LaGrange, IL 60525
Toll-free (877) Spine Dr
www.spine.org

Introduction, *iii*

Dedicated to my three best friends:
Gayle, Aaron and Hannah

The Couch Potato Workout

Introduction

You are probably
wondering why anyone would
write a book about exercises
for couch potatoes. The point
is, these exercises can be done
anywhere you are, without
special equipment or a large
time commitment. You don't
have to make major changes
to your lifestyle to enjoy

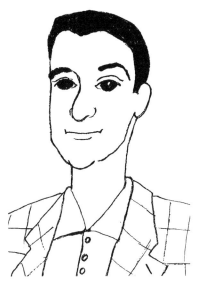

increased physical fitness and a greater sense of well
being. Even if you are really lazy, this book can show
you simple strengthening techniques you can easily
incorporate into your everyday routine.

This book describes numerous practical
and functional exercises you can do without large
amounts of time spent on preparation and execution.
Everyone is busy and has a hard time finding the
time to do exercises for the many physical problems
we face or simply to stay in better shape (for those
lucky enough not to have significant sports, work or
musculoskeletal aches and pains.) These 101 exercises
can be integrated into your normal day. In fact, all
of the exercises in this book are meant to be done as

part of your daily activities. We have incorporated a component or two of exercise into every day tasks for those times you can't go to the gym or keep specific time in your day to do your exercise program.

The exercises we have chosen are meant to be functional, meaning they work a specific body part in a manner resembling how that body part normally functions each day. You will notice that many of the exercises in this book are done in a standing position. Most of what we do all day long requires us to be on our feet. Many exercises are done on one leg at a time because walking is done one leg at a time. One-legged exercises simulate what your bones and muscles do when you walk. Standing on one leg at a time also requires a great deal of balance. Improving balance is an important component of many sports-specific activities, as well as a good way to prevent falls that can break a hip. For example, changing directions on one leg after hitting a tennis shot or landing on one foot playing basketball are examples of the importance of balance in sports. Even catching your balance after tripping on a rock or a curb are examples of the importance of balance for everyone.

Another important aspect about functional exercises (in addition to simulating our sporting or daily activities and improving balance) is that they focus on all the different directions in which we move. You may have been instructed to do a hamstring stretch where you straighten you leg and lean toward your toes. In fact, with that stretch you are only stretching the hamstring in one plane of motion. If you turn your foot in and out when you do that stretch you will stretch the hamstring in three different planes of motion, all directions for which you may have to move that muscle when you walk, turn around, get in and out of a car or the shower. In other words, muscles and joints need to be exercised in different planes, or directions, in order to prepare them for all of the activities that we do.

This book is organized by body part. Exercises are described that primarily emphasize that specific body part. However, as we know, the musculoskeletal system is a complex system of many bones, joint and muscles interconnected in kinetic (movement) chains. These kinetic chains require many different and often distant muscles to work together to accomplish a task. For example, standing and shaving requires many lower extremity muscles to support our body while our upper back muscles support our arms to stabilize our hands and wrists so we can shave. Therefore, many exercises can be cross-referenced to other areas that are also worked with that specific exercise.

All exercises in this book were selected because they are part of some activity of daily living. These are not home exercises that require a specific time allotted for exercise. These are exercises that are already part of what you are doing each day. We have developed exercises for every room in the house, every time of the day, every different activity that you may do.

Over the last decade or more, the health care

professionals at the Sports Rehabilitation Program of the Rehabilitation Institute of Chicago have integrated these exercises into our patients' home programs. When the exercise takes very little time, when it is an extension of things you are doing anyway, when they are very functional in their nature, and most of all, fun to do, compliance is very high. The benefit of the exercises is also therefore quite high.

Although this book does not present a comprehensive exercise program, it is a great way for people to stay fit and healthy and address some of their musculoskeletal maladies, even if they never leave the couch!

About the North American Spine Society

The North American Spine Society (NASS) is a multidisciplinary medical organization dedicated to advancing quality spine care through education, research and advocacy. Since its start in 1985, NASS has grown to over 4,000 member health care professionals in 22 spine-related specialties.

- The NASS Annual Meeting provides education to health care professional on the latest spine care research findings and treatment developments.

- *The Spine Journal*, NASS' peer-reviewed medical journal, was recognized for its unique contribution to the field by acceptance into *Index Medicus/* MEDLINE in its second year of publication.

- NASS' Research Grants and Fellowships program supports the best spine research and has provided over $2 million in research funding to date.

- NASS is committed to advocating on behalf of its members and patients for access to spine care.

- *Spine Health* is NASS' annual public education campaign to raise awareness of spine health maintenance and the impact of spine problems on society. More information about spine disorders and treatment options can be found on the NASS Web site, www.spine.org.

About the Rehabilitation Institute of Chicago

Founded in 1954, the Rehabilitation Institute of Chicago (RIC) has earned a worldwide reputation as a leader in patient care, advocacy, research and educating health professionals in physical medicine and rehabilitation. People from around the globe choose RIC because of our expertise in treating a range of conditions, from the most complex conditions including cerebral palsy, spinal cord injury, stroke and traumatic brain injury, to the more common, such as arthritis, chronic pain and sports injuries. RIC has been recognized as the "Best Rehabilitation Hospital in America" every year since 1991 by *U.S. News & World Report*.

- RIC has over 30 locations in the Chicago area and southern Illinois.

- RIC offers programs and services to improve the quality of life for people with physical disabilities.

- RIC is the home of the Northwestern University Feinberg School of Medicine's Department of Physical Medicine and Rehabilitation.

- Searle Research Center at RIC is one of the largest programs of its kind in the country, attracting research scientists from around the globe and more than $6 million in federal and private foundation grants and other donations.

Chapter 1 - Head and Neck

Our heads weigh roughly eight to ten pounds (depending on what's in there!) Our head should sit pretty well centered on our neck and shoulders so the muscles of the neck and upper back don't have to work too hard. With the exception of ballet dancers, most of us have "average lousy" posture where the head seems to be a little bit (or a lot) in front of the rest of our body. Most of us can look sideways in a mirror and notice that "hunched forward" look. It places additional stress on the upper back and forces neck muscles to work extra hard to hold the 8-10 pound object back over the rest of the body so it doesn't tip forward. Thus the upper back and neck muscles get fatigued and often tighten up. Many of the exercises in this section are aimed at improving "average lousy" posture and strengthening the upper back and neck. An added advantage is that your mother won't bother you as much to sit or stand up straight.

Neck muscles have a tendency to become stiff and achy from prolonged periods of sitting at desks and in cars, so we have also added a number of flexibility exercises that may help relieve some to these symptoms.

Exercise #1 - Wall Angels

As a kid most of us were familiar with making "angels in the snow" where we lie in a fresh patch of snow and move our arms up and down. "Wall angels" are performed standing up against a wall. Typically, your feet may be two to three inches from the wall. Your buttocks, shoulder blades, and back of the head should be aligned against the wall. The chin should be tucked with the head 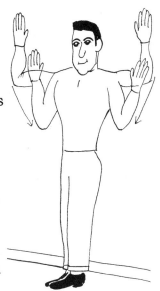 against the wall so you don't simply arch your neck backwards to be able to touch the wall. You should think about tucking your chin, and even making a double chin, to keep your head and neck in the right position. Put your arms against the wall with the elbows bent (almost like a "stick up") position. Do the best you can about keeping your elbows, forearms and hands against the wall. Finally, imagine putting your elbows in your back pockets. Obviously, you cannot actually get your elbows in your back pockets, but that is the motion you want to try to accomplish for this exercises to be most useful. Pulling your elbows back and down ("into your back pockets") allows you to work important postural muscles (your middle and lower trapezii, for the technically inclined) and not work your upper back muscles (upper trapezius) as much. Most of us have way too much activity in our upper trapezius muscles due to tension from sitting at desks and driving in cars.

The object of this exercise is to hold the "wall angel" position with your elbows in your pockets for 20 to 30 seconds against the wall. Make sure you continue to breathe normally! After finishing, you feel your posture is a little more upright. This can be done as many times during the day as you have time. We recommend you do it at least two to three times a day. It only will take up 90 seconds of time and will improve your posture, decrease tension in your upper back, and particularly for post-menopausal women, help combat some of the potential postural changes that can occur with osteoporosis.

Exercise 2 - Elbows Down, Chest Out ("Stick 'Em Down!")

This exercise is excellent for breaking up that hunched forward, head forward, slouched posture that we have all acquired since our descent from apes and then de-evolved through sitting at desks, working on computers and sitting in cars in traffic. This exercise is done by sitting up straight wherever it is that we are sitting. Specifically we try to push our chest out about one inch or so in order to have our chest in front of our face. You put both arms down to the side, with the palms facing forward, and try to push the arms gently toward the floor while maintaining the chest out position. At the same time spread your fingers apart as far as they will go for 8 to 10 seconds. Then relax and repeat a few times. You should feel a pleasant stretch across your chest and arms, forearms and fingers.

Exercise #3 - Head Rest Slide

This exercise improves posture and decreases the work to the neck muscles. While sitting in a **stationary** car, press the back of your head against the head rest and try to slowly raise your head up against the headrest with your head in constant contact with the head rest. When you get it up as high as you can, hold it there for five seconds then relax. You can repeat this five or six times.

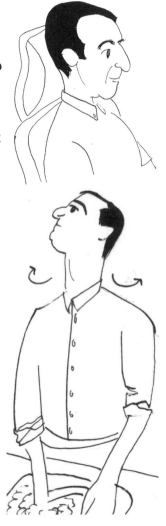

Exercise #4 - Doing the Dishes Neck Circles

This exercise is easily done while doing the always fun task of washing the dishes. As you are standing there at the sink,

slowly rotate your neck in a clockwise position trying to extend the tip of your head out as far as possible. After three or four rotations, repeat the exercise in a counter-clockwise position. Remember these rotations should be done **slowly** and in a pain free range of motion. Besides increasing the flexibility of the neck, these exercises can pass the time of doing dishes.

Exercise #5 - Shower Neck Stretch

This is the same exercise as #4 but can be done in the shower with warm water flowing across your neck, or while singing in the shower.

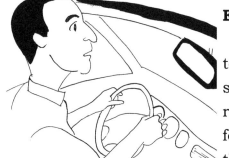

Exercise #6 - Mirror Look

An interesting way to work on sitting up straight without trying to remember to do three or four things at once is to do the "Mirror Look." When you get into your car to drive, tilt the mirror up slightly higher than what you normally would put it. As you back out of the driveway or garage, force yourself to sit up straighter to look out the mirror rather than lowering it. You may want to start with this exercise just for brief periods to get used to improved posture.

Exercises #7 and #8 and #9 - "Don't move the Razor/ Brush/Facial Cream" Exercises

These exercises help to increase the range of

motion of the neck. All of these address neck range of motion in multiple different planes of movement, which is important since we ask our necks to move in many different directions all day long (i.e., looking down at the floor, over our shoulders when we

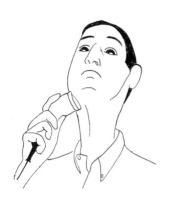

drive and side to side in conversation).

When shaving with an electric razor, most men move the shaver in all directions as the head and face are held still. With this exercise the shaver is held in one position and the face (and therefore neck) is moved. With this type of motion, the neck is moved in many different directions to increase flexibility. A variation of this exercise for both men and women is to do the same thing with a toothbrush. In other words, hold the toothbrush in one place and move your mouth and teeth around for your dental care. Since brushing your teeth may be done more vigorously than shaving, this variation of the exercise actually strengthens some of the neck muscles also.

A last variation of this exercise for women who put on facial cream is to hold the cream in one hand and move the face around to put on the cream. A higher level skill related to this would be putting on mascara by holding the mascara stick and

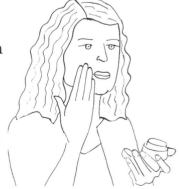

moving the eyelashes to put on the mascara rather than holding the face still and moving the hands and wrist.

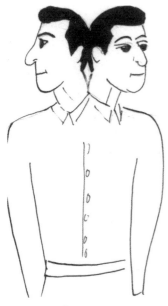

Exercise #10 - Reading the Paper

This is another exercise where cervical motion is substituted for movement, this time eye movement. When reading the newspaper, instead of moving from line to line using your eye muscles, slowly move your neck from side to side to gently stretch your neck muscles.

Exercise #11 - Street Cross

Similar to #10, when you are about to cross the street walking, or making a turn while driving, rotate the head as far as you can in both directions first. Besides looking both ways before you cross the street, you can also give the muscles of your neck a gentle stretch. Your mother would be pleased.

Exercise #12 - Escalator Gaze

This exercise provides a slightly larger range of motion in turning the head and neck sideways. It actually starts to bring in some of the rotational motion of the thoracic or mid back region. When going up (or down) an escalator, focus on an object or person going the opposite direction on the escalator. Follow that object or person until you get to the top or bottom of the escalator. Try not to turn at the hips, knees or ankles when you do this exercise to get a better mid back and neck stretch.

Chapter 2 - Shoulders

The shoulder joint has a tremendous amount of mobility when it works properly. In other words, we can move it in many directions. When we have injuries to the ligaments (i.e., after a fall) or to the muscles and tendons (i.e., throwing baseballs and other types of overuse problems affecting the rotator cuff muscles) mobility of the shoulder can be decreased. Therefore, a number of exercises in this section address range of motion exercises for the shoulder that can be done with your daily activities.

To strengthen muscles around the shoulder in a functional way, we emphasize motions that simulate how the shoulder really works. For instance, instead of keeping the elbow against the side of your body and rotating your arm outward (which doesn't look much like any activity most of us do in our daily lives) emphasis is placed on diagonal type motions. These are movements that move from one spot on one side of the body to another location on the other side of the body in a direction that we typically would perform. We can strengthen the shoulder by adding resistance or weight (in the form of milk!)

Exercise #13 - Diagonal Window Washing

When washing windows or squeegeeing the shower, you can move your shoulder through what are called diagonal planes to increase the range of motion of the shoulder. These diagonal motions start by reaching up over your opposite shoulder and pulling down and across your body to an area near your knees. The internal

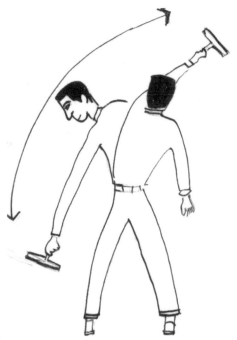

and external rotation movements that occur can help shoulder flexibility.

Exercise #14 - Back Scrub

Another good shoulder range of motion exercise for the shower is scrubbing your back with a wash cloth or soap. Reach behind your back with each arm and then raise your hand up your back as far as it will go (without a lot of pain!). This exercise is more advanced than Diagonal Window Washing because more shoulder rotation is required.

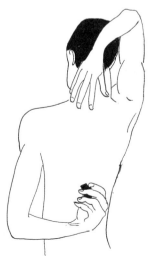

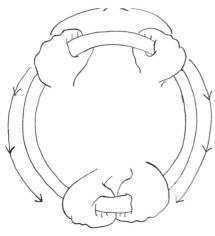

Exercise #15 - Steering Wheel Roll

This exercise is a gentle one for shoulder mobility. While stopped at a stop light, or waiting in a parked car (never do this while driving!), take your hands from the proper "ten and two" position and slowly take your left hand and move clockwise around the steering wheel while you move your right hand counter clockwise around the steering wheel until the two hands meet at the bottom of the steering wheel. Then return back going the opposite direction with each hand to the previous "ten and two" position.

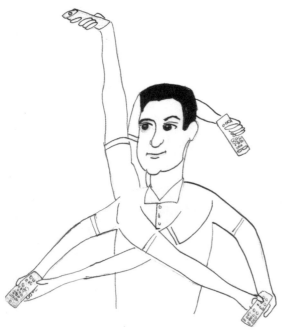

Exercise #16 - Remote Shuffle

This is the perfect exercise for anyone who loves watching football on a Sunday afternoon, commands the remote control, has a satellite dish with ten or more games on at once and likes to watch all the games and not miss a play. The objective is to click the remote in a different place in space each time you change channels. You should try to reach out as far as you can each time you click the remote including over your head, across your body, behind your back etc. This exercise can be done with both hands to maximize shoulder mobility. The additional benefit is strengthening of the muscles that flex the thumb.

Exercise #17 - "El Train" Stretch
Beginner

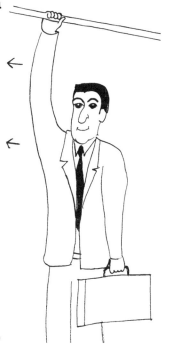

That's Subway (Elevated or "El") Train Stretch, for all you non-Chicagoans. Ideally, you'll want to do this stretch on the train when you have to stand because no seats are available. But do it when the train is not packed with people, since these motions on a crowded train may get you arrested. While holding on to the overhead rail slowly lean your body toward the arm you are holding up. Hold the stretch for 20 to 30 seconds. You should feel a gentle stretch under your arms. Repeat this three or four times, if it's not too crowded. Make sure you hold on tightly to avoid falling in to an unsuspecting person's lap.

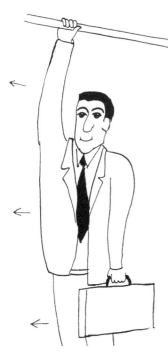

Exercise #18 - El Train Stretch Advanced

The advanced stretch allows you to get a good side stretch too. Again this stretch can only be done on a relatively bare train. Lean your entire body toward the direction of your hanging arm. Be careful to maintain your feet on the ground to maintain the sustained stretch. Again, hold the stretch for 20 to 30 seconds at a time.

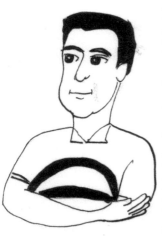

Exercise #19 - Steering Wheel Hug

This exercise is for those times when you are stopped in traffic, and you can feel all that stress from a long, difficult day in your upper back and neck, and just need to stretch out a little. Reach around and gently hug the steering wheel. It doesn't have to be firm (remember this is only a steering wheel, not a loved one). Once this is done, gently lower your mid back toward the back of the car seat. You should feel a gentle stretch between your shoulder blades that helps to relax those tight muscles.

Exercise #20 - Milk Carton Lifts

Start with a partially filled milk carton. With the carton in your right hand about waist level, lift the carton toward your left shoulder. Then take it back down to your right side. You can then lift it over your head on the right (keep the cap on to avoid making a mess) and then across your body to waist height on the left side. This sequence can be repeated a few times. As strength and flexibility improve, you will be able to lift a fuller carton of milk and raise and lower the carton to higher and lower levels.

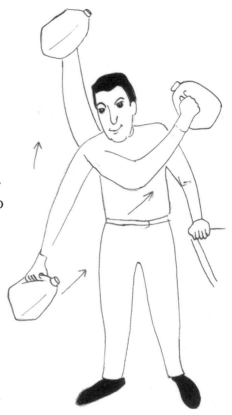

Exercise # 21 - Milk Carton Stretch

This exercise is a good one for people who get generalized stiffness in their shoulder joint (the ball and socket joint) or a "frozen" shoulder. You can take the same milk carton from the refrigerator and hold it dangling down in your hand with your other arm supporting you against a counter and leaning over slightly forward. Slowly rotate the carton in small

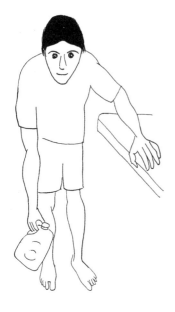

circles starting in one direction and slowly increasing the diameter of the circles. Then slowly change the direction you are turning first with large circles then moving to smaller circles. This maneuver can be done one or two times to feel a good stretch around the shoulder girdle.

Exercise #22 - Brief Case Lifts

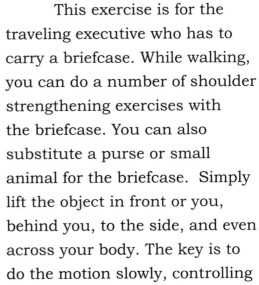

This exercise is for the traveling executive who has to carry a briefcase. While walking, you can do a number of shoulder strengthening exercises with the briefcase. You can also substitute a purse or small animal for the briefcase. Simply lift the object in front or you, behind you, to the side, and even across your body. The key is to do the motion slowly, controlling the lifting up and slowly lowering it down. You do not want this to be a rapid-fire motion, which can injure the shoulder. This exercise can be done standing in the elevator (even done on one leg when no one is looking for additional balance training), walking down the street or while waiting at a bus stop.

Exercise #23 - OJ Range of Motion Shake

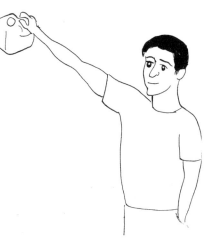

This exercise will strengthen the shoulder girdle muscles through small movements back and forth at the shoulder with some light weights (in this case a carton of orange juice). Take an almost empty half gallon carton of orange juice and raise it over your head; then slowly lower it down to your side while shaking the orange juice carton as you would before you poured a glass to drink. This motion can be repeated many times in different directions to increase range of motion around the shoulder and strengthen the shoulder in different planes. Increase the amount of liquid in the carton as your shoulder becomes stronger.

Chapter 3 - Elbows

Many of the exercises that work the muscles around the elbow actually are done to help with wrist and hand motions. The muscles around the elbow are the prime movers of the wrist and hand.

Exercises #27 through #32 are excellent for wrist and hand dexterity and mobility. They can also be done at home or at your local pub. These exercises were first perfected by a number of our staff members who were diligently thinking about work and new exercises for our patients one Friday afternoon at a local drinking establishment.

Exercise #24 - Remote Wrist Lifts

This exercise is a distant cousin of Exercise #16. It can also be done on any Sunday afternoon watching multiple football games. Simply take the remote control (use the biggest one you have from the pile of remotes) and, while sitting watching your favorite team or movie and your arm pointing toward the TV, aim the remote at the ceiling moving your wrist only. Hold it there for 10 seconds then aim it at the floor, again only moving the wrist. Repeat this three to four times during every commercial. Be careful not to accidentally change the channel when doing this exercise or it may irritate people who are watching TV with you.

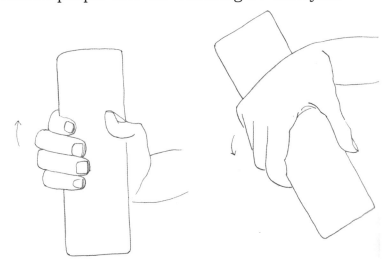

Exercise 25 - Double Lift

If you happen to have a second remote (and who doesn't?), you can lift both objects (one in each hand) in the same direction each time you change the channel. Just don't press the buttons on the second remote to avoid messing up the channels and/or TV reception. This is an advanced version of #24.

Exercise 26 - Lift and Hold

This even more highly advanced version of #24 and #25 requires you to hold the remote control (and

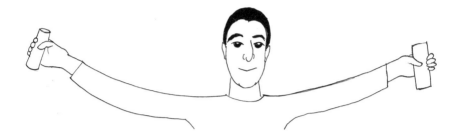

a beverage for a real challenge) in place in some point in space for the duration of the commercial(s) you're watching. This can be very challenging during a World Series or Super Bowl game with extended commercial coverage.

Exercise #27 - Coaster Flip

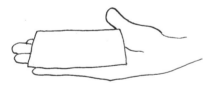

The first basic exercise is to take a coaster, preferably one of heavier type paper or cardboard, put it about half hanging over the edge of a table and flip the coaster into the air with your index finger and then catch the coaster with your palm up.

Exercise #28 - Coaster Flip with Pinch

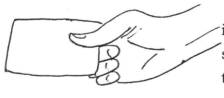

The next exercise in this series is done similarly to #27 except that after you flip the coaster in the air you try to catch the coaster between your thumb and your index finger with a "pinch" grasp.

Exercise #29 - Multiple Coaster Flip

Another variation is to flip two coasters, one with each hand and catch them with the palms of both hands.

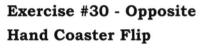

Exercise #30 - Opposite Hand Coaster Flip

Try the coaster flip exercise with your non-dominant hand (or the one you don't write or throw a ball with.) You can try catching the coaster first with your dominant hand and then with your non-dominant hand.

Exercise #31 - Bilateral Coaster Flip with Pinch

Flip two coasters at once and catch them with a pinch grip (like # 28).

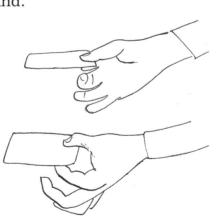

Exercise #32 - Eyes Closed Multiple Coaster Flip

This is one for the experienced coaster flipper only. Try flipping both coasters with your eyes closed and catching them in your palms.

Chapter 4 - Wrist/Hand

Wrist and hand exercises can be done almost anywhere and with little equipment or props. Dexterity and coordination are two functions of the hands and fingers that can be trained, especially when you ask your non-dominant hand to perform functions that are normally done by your dominant hand. This can be useful, particularly for sports that require two hands for use (i.e., basketball, baseball) as well as promoting the use of both hands for daily activities like trimming bushes and washing windows.

Exercise #33 - Opposite Hand Cereal Feed

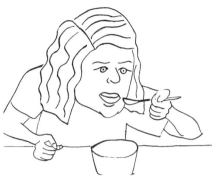

Eat your cereal in the morning using your non-dominant hand. When you first try this, put a napkin over your tie or over your lap. Trust me on this.

Exercise #34 - Opposite Hand Cereal Feed, Eyes Closed

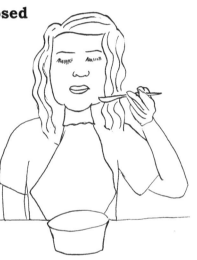

This one really requires extra napkins or towels over your clothes before trying. Besides working on hand coordination, this exercise challenges your sense of position and where your limbs are in space.

Exercise #35 - Finger Hair Wash

This is still another simple exercise to do in the shower. When washing your hair, use the tips of your fingers to scrub your scalp rather than emphasizing arm and forearm motion.

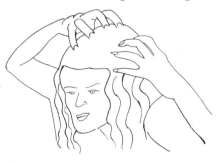

Besides strengthening the finger flexor and extensor muscles, you will probably do a better job of cleaning your scalp.

Exercise #36 - Boring Meeting Hand Stretch

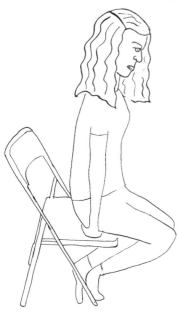

Another way to stretch the wrist muscles and tendons (the ones that flex and extend the wrist joint) is to sit on your hands with the palms up or palms down for a few seconds at a time. This can be done during a boring meeting, car ride, etc. Simply place your hands, either palm down or palm up right under your gluteal muscles (that's your buttocks!) and slowly straighten out your elbows until you feel a gentle stretch in your forearms. Hold this for 15 to 20 seconds and then repeat 3 or 4 times. This stretch has the added advantage of warming your hands on a cold day such as at sporting events outside in fall and winter.

Exercise #37 - Sink Wrist Stretch

Another way to stretch the wrist flexor muscles and tendons is to put your palms down on the sink in the morning and slowly lean forward, putting a slight stretch on the wrist and forearm muscles. To stretch the wrist extensors put the back of your hands on the sink, keep the elbows straight and slightly lean forward to get the forearm stretch.

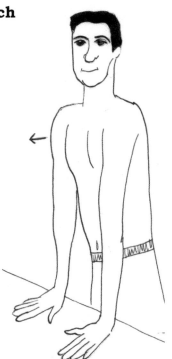

Chapter 5 - Upper Back

The upper back needs to be strong to support the shoulders, arms and head. It is also a crucial area for proper posture which, if optimal (or at least decent), can decrease the stress on the cervical spine (neck region) and head. Most exercises in this book will emphasize strengthening of the interscapular (between the shoulder blades) muscles (i.e., the middle and lower trapezii, and spine extensors).

The Door Jamb Series (exercises #43 through #45) stretches out the chest muscles, the upper back, shoulders and hips. All they require is a door jamb. Chances are you will have to go through a few doors during your daily activities. These exercises can be done at any time and only take a few seconds each to get a good stretch and, in some cases, work on strength and balance.

Exercise #38 - Pillow Head Raise

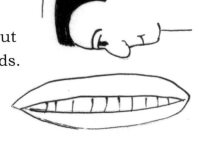

When laying in bed with your face down, slowly raise your head off the pillow without extending your neck backwards. You may need to concentrate on keeping your chin tucked in while you do this to avoid arching your head backwards. Once you lift your head up, hold it five to 10 seconds, relax and repeat three or four times.

Exercise #39 - Towel Dry Off

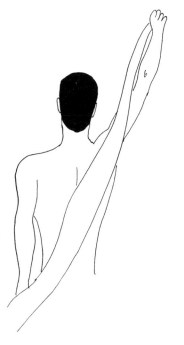

This exercise is the first of a trio of exercises that get you to pull your shoulder blades back and stretch out your chest (pectoral) muscles. The chest muscles often get very tight from sitting at computers and driving in cars all day. Take a large shower towel and put it behind your back and proceed to dry off your back by moving your arms in a back and forth motion. This can be done with both arms at the side or with one arm above your shoulder and one down by your waist. Alternate positions of both arms while drying off your back.

Exercise #40 - Towel Dry Off Intermediate

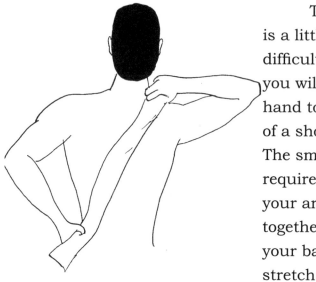

This exercise is a little more difficult because you will now use a hand towel instead of a shower towel. The smaller towel requires you to put your arms closer together behind your back and thus stretch out your chest muscles and strengthen your mid back muscles.

Exercise #41 - Towel Dry Off Advanced

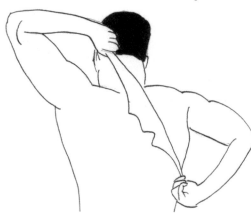

This is the tough one. Perform the same type of motion using a small wash cloth. You need greater range of motion at the shoulders and the ability to pull your shoulders back even further. This exercise may require more time to dry yourself off, so it may be more difficult during winter months in northern cities or with lousy heating.

Exercise #42 - Towel Dry with a Stretch

Do this exercise after you have finished drying off and want a good stretch for your upper back and chest muscles. The towel gives you a more pronounced, effective stretch. Take the towel behind your back, hold the towel stretched out as far as it will go, and pull your hands toward the floor while standing up straight. Hold this stretch for 5-10 seconds and repeat a few times. You should feel your chest press out, your shoulder blades retract (or pull backwards) and it possibly could be easier to take a big breath.

Exercise #43 - Door Jamb Pec Stretch

This exercise, as its name implies, stretches the pectorals or front chest muscles. Many of us have that hunched forward posture from gravity and sitting at desks and in cars all day which causes our chest muscles to get tighter which further accentuates our "average lousy" posture. The pec stretch is done simply by standing in the door jamb, putting your arms up along the sides of the door jamb and

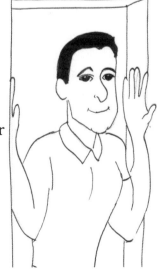

slowly leaning forward (using the palms of your hands to hold on) as you gently stretch your chest muscles. This exercise can be held for 5-10 seconds at a time, then repeated 3-4 times.

Exercise #44 - Door Jamb with a Twist

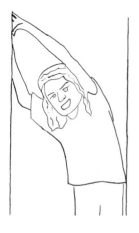

This exercise can stretch some of your side muscles and shoulder muscles and can be especially helpful before playing sports like tennis or baseball that require twisting the mid and lower back and shoulder flexibility. Instead of putting your arms overhead, put both hands on one side of the door jamb at head or shoulder level and lean sideways. You should feel your body tugging gently along your side muscles and back of the shoulder.

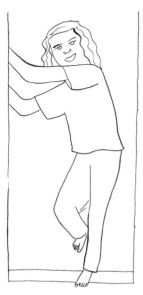

Exercise #45 - One Legged Door Jamb with a Twist

To add some balance and strength exercises to the door jamb series, you can try doing exercise #44 on one leg. This will challenge your balance and strengthen your hip muscles at the same time as stretching some back muscles.

Chapter 6 – Lower Back

Low back pain is quite common for all of us. Often we are given sheets and sheets of exercises by our health care providers and cannot find much time to take time out from our busy schedules to do all those exercises.

These exercises are geared to strengthening many of the back, hip and lower extremity muscles that are important in protecting our back from the many physical stresses that are applied to them every day. We have tried to make these exercises fun, easy to do and closely resemble the way your body has to move to perform many of your daily activities.

Exercise #46 - Rake (or Sweep) and Twist

This exercise is done while raking the leaves or sweeping the floor. The key is to take long strokes with the rake and turn at your hips as you rake the leaves toward you. This exercise should be done in both directions (i.e. going from left to right and right to left). Make sure that you turn at the hips and back and not make your arms do all the work.

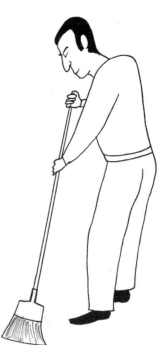

Exercise #47 - Put the Dishes Away Twist

Similar to the Rake and Twist, this exercise requires that you turn your body from side to side while allowing motion to occur at the hips and back.

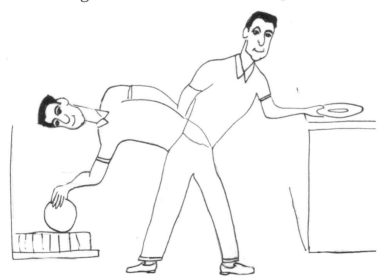

This exercise can be done as you take the dishes out of the dishwasher (usually at a lower level) and then putting the dishes on the shelf (usually at a higher level). It is useful to put the dishes and silverware away one item at a time to get more out of this exercise. This may even add a little interest to a fairly mundane activity.

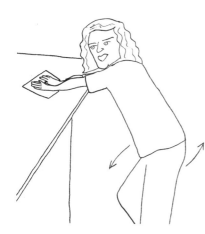

Exercise #48 - Cleaning the Counter Top Swivel

This exercise is also a variation of #46 and #47. While cleaning off the table after a meal, make sure you add the hip and back motion to the cleaning movements of your hand instead of simply using your hand, elbow and shoulder to do all the work. This may look a little funny (kind of like dancing) to those who have not read this book but it will help with hip, pelvic and back motion and still get the counter clean.

Exercise #49 - Laundry Toss

This exercise will work the abdominal muscles, low back muscles and hip muscles in a rotational movement. It will also make doing the laundry more interesting. Stand 10 to 15 feet away from the washing machine. Put the dirty laundry basket on your left side. The washing machine should be on your right

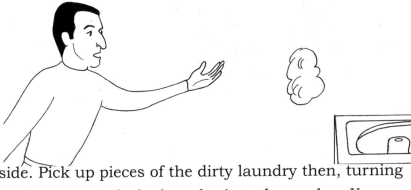

side. Pick up pieces of the dirty laundry then, turning at the hips, pitch the laundry into the washer. You may have to pick up some of the laundry that misses the target. Once you've mastered the dry laundry, you can move on to throwing wet laundry from the washer into the dryer.

Exercise #50 - Overhead Laundry Toss

This is a progression from #49 and adds a different plane of motion. Put the laundry basket directly in front of you and have the washer or dryer directly behind you. Grab a piece or two of dirty clothes, reach over your head slowly and drop the laundry into the washer.

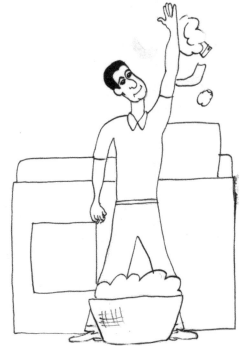

Again, start with dry clothes then progress to wet clothes from the washer into the dryer.

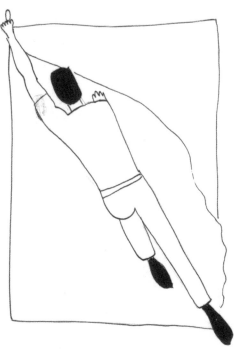

Exercise #51 - Tuck the Corners on All Fours

This exercise incorporates a beginning stabilization exercise for the core muscles (i.e., back, side, abdominal, hip muscles) into making your bed. On your hands and knees, extend one leg out and use the opposite hand to tuck in the corners of your sheets when making the bed.

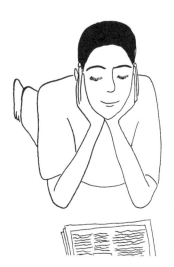

Exercise #52 - Arched Reading

Many people spend a great amount of time during their day flexed forward sitting at desks, in cars, on trains, and at computers. To balance this falling forward posture we develop, try reading or watching TV on your stomach with your back arched, propped up on your elbows.

Exercise #53 – Latte Dance

Do this exercise at the kitchen counter as

you prepare your coffee. The goal is to stand on one leg and rotate right and left rather than stepping as you reach for the coffee can, cup and pot.

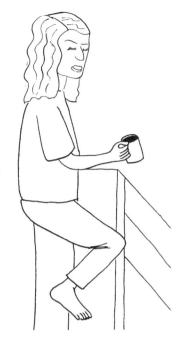

Exercise #54 - Underarm Wash

This is a great exercise to stretch and strengthen some of your side muscles (quadratus lumborum for the anatomically interested) that support your lumbar spine. It also makes you smell better. In the shower, tilt your hips to the left while you take your left arm and reach overhead and over your right shoulder as far as you can comfortably lean. Hold this position for 5 to 10 seconds while you wash under your left arm. You should feel a stretch along your side as you reach as far as you can. By slowly returning to an upright position, and then leaning and stretching to the other side, you can actually do some strengthening of these muscles, too.

Exercise #55 - Underarm Wash with a Twist

To add a different plane of motion to exercise

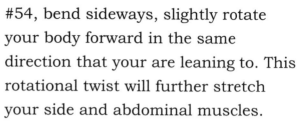

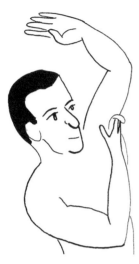

#54, bend sideways, slightly rotate your body forward in the same direction that your are leaning to. This rotational twist will further stretch your side and abdominal muscles.

Exercise #56 - Standing Side Stretch

While standing up straight, with some weighted object in either hand (i.e., a briefcase, carton of milk, the garbage) slowly lower the hand with the weight in it as far as down your side it will go. This exercise will stretch your side muscles. Hold it there for 15 to 20 seconds. Then put the weighted object in the opposite hand and repeat. The heavier the object the more stretch your will place on the side muscles.

Exercise #57 - Lying Down Side Stretch (*illustration, top of next page*)

Do this exercise when you are watching TV on the couch and want to get in a little stretching, particularly for your side muscles. While lying on your side, prop your arm up on the arm rest or end of the couch with your hand supporting your head. Slowly lower your side into the couch with the weight of your body feeling a stretch on your side muscles. Shift to the other side of the couch to stretch the opposite side.

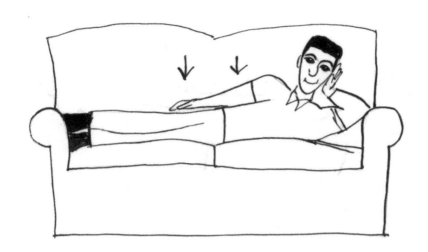

Exercise #58 - Sideways TV Watch

After stretching your side muscles with exercise #57, use the following exercise to strengthen them. While watching TV, lay on your side, prop up on your elbow, then straighten your body. Hold this position for at least 10 to 15 seconds.

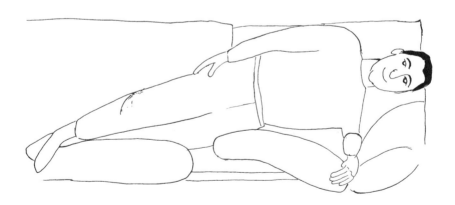

Exercise #59 - Cheetos® Stretch

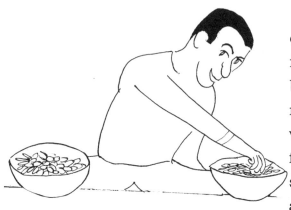

This is an excellent exercise for stretching the back and shoulder muscles while watching your favorite television show and having a little snack. Place two bowls of chips or other treats on the table in front of you far enough away that you have to reach for them. Eat the treats (pretzels, potato chips, or cut up vegetables work well here) one at a time. Start by reaching with your right hand into the bowl on the left side of the table. Take only one piece of food or one snack at a time to increase the number of repetitions. Then reach with your left hand to the bowl on the right. Repeat as dictated by hunger or amount of food available.

Exercise #60 - Cheetos® Twist with a Dip

This is the same as #59 except that you put a container of chip dip on the floor between the two bowls and dip the chips one at a time after reaching across your body to get the potato chip or vegetable. This exercise adds some wrist rotation to the shoulder and back motion of Exercise #59.

Chapter 7 - Hip and Pelvis

The hip and pelvis are the base of the support for the low back as well as the base of support for all our lower extremity muscles and joints. If things are not right at the base, then all those structures below and above cannot function optimally. We spend a great deal of time teaching patients how to improve their core strength, which includes the hip and pelvic muscles, along with their spinal and lower limb muscles.

Another very important part of musculoskeletal rehabilitation of spine and sports injuries is balance and what is called proprioceptive training. Proprioception is the ability to know where your body is in space. When we jump in the air and land, the ability to land softly is driven to some extent by proprioception. Proprioception can be thought of as a combination of balance and agility. Many of the exercises in this section are excellent for a variety of musculoskeletal disorders as well as for enhancing functional movements and sports.

The next few exercises are some of the easiest to integrate into your daily routine and some of the best at improving lower limb balance, strength and proprioception.

Exercise #61 - Toothbrush Series

This is the first in a series of the trademark exercises of this book. Stand on one leg while holding on to the counter as you brush your teeth. You should brush for at least two to three minutes.

Exercise #62 - Toothbrush, No Holding

The next progression of this series is to brush your teeth standing on one leg without holding on. Alternate one leg then the other each time you brush your teeth. Also try brushing with your nondominant hand (the one you don't write or throw a ball with).

Exercise #63 - Toothbrush, Eyes Closed

Now perform the exercise without holding on with both eyes closed. This is easily done with the lights on or off, thereby conserving energy.

Exercise #64 - Toothbrush, Head Move

Next, without holding on, on one leg, move your head instead of your toothbrush to clean all your teeth. In this way you are adding cervical motion to your standing balance exercise.

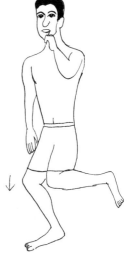

Exercise #65 - Toothbrush, Knees Bent

This exercise is done while standing on one leg and bending your knee as far down as you can get and maintain your balance. When you've mastered this exercise, try it with your eyes closed. To add more function to this exercise, try bending your knees as you lean in different directions (i.e., forward, backwards, to each side).

Exercise #66 - Toothbrush with a Hop

This advanced level exercise is done while brushing your teeth on one leg and hopping.

Exercise #67 - One Leg Flossing

As the name implies, simply stand on one leg while flossing. The back and forth action of the flossing will add balance and agility training to simply standing on one leg.

Exercise #68 - Elevator Hamstring Stretch

This exercise can be done in an elevator that has any kind of railing in it. It will usually need to be

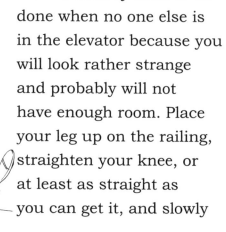

done when no one else is in the elevator because you will look rather strange and probably will not have enough room. Place your leg up on the railing, straighten your knee, or at least as straight as you can get it, and slowly lean forward with your chest out. Don't bend over at your back. This exercise is meant to stretch your hamstring not increase the stress on your low back. Try this stretch in three different positions: the leg straight, slightly turned in and slightly turned out. These variations allow you to stretch the hamstrings in different planes of motion.

Exercise #69 - Foot Wash/Dry

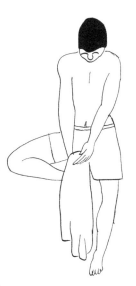

This exercise also builds balance and coordination. While drying off your feet after a shower or bath, try drying the foot and leg while standing on the other leg. A variation of this exercise is to wash your feet in the shower while standing on one leg. You need to have secure footing on your balance leg to do this exercise safely.

Exercise #70 - Toilet Hamstring Stretch

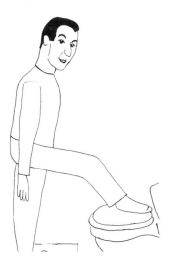

This exercise is similar to the elevator stretch but done in the bathroom after a shower. The height of the toilet is probably a little lower than the railing in the elevator, and the bathroom is usually less crowded. This exercise is also done with the leg straight or slightly bent, then slightly turned in, then slightly turned out. Again, emphasis is placed on keeping your chest in front of your face to put the stretch on your hamstring and not your back.

Exercise #71 - Sink Hamstring Stretch

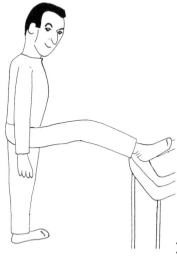

This exercise is the advanced version of #70. After you have mastered the stretch at toilet level, you can then lift your leg to the sink and perform the same stretch.

Exercise #72 - Escalator Stretch

If you live in a building or frequent a mall that has an escalator, this exercise will stretch your hip flexor muscles and your calf muscles. While going up the escalator, put your left foot on a step and bend that same knee as much as possible; keep it comfortable. At the same time take your right leg and extend it back as far as you can to a lower step.

Try to keep both feet flat on the their respective steps. Try to reach back to as low a step as possible to get the greatest amount of stretch. Then simply ride the escalator to the next level.

Exercise #73 - Escalator/Groin Stretch

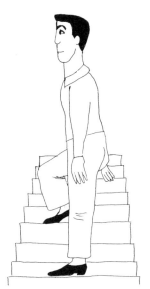

To stretch the adductors or groin muscles, stagger your legs on two different steps, either one or two steps away from each other. Face your body directly to the other escalator (assuming one is there). Lean your body slowly to the right, then to the left to get a gentle groin stretch.

Exercise #74 - Escalator with a Twist

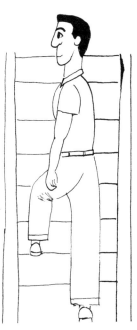

On either one of the two previous exercises, in order to get some stretch through the low and mid back, slowly turn your entire body to the left and to the right (i.e., gazing over your shoulder).

Exercise #75 Toilet Hip Flexor Stretch

The hip flexor muscles are quite strong and have a tendency to

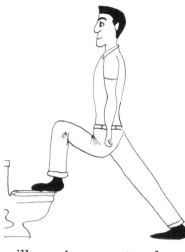

get very tight, especially from sitting too much, which puts them in a shortened position. Either before or after using the toilet (preferably after), put the seat down and close the lid, putting one leg up on the toilet lid. With this knee bent, reach back with the opposite leg as far as it will go. As you stand up straight and then bend down again you should feel a stretch on the front part of the hip or hip flexor of the leg that is on the ground. Repeat on both sides.

Exercise #76 - One Legged Dressing

A simple way to do one leg standing exercises is to put your socks and shoes on while standing on one leg at a time. This requires use of the hands, wrists and fingers, in coordination with lower limb balance.

Exercise #77 - Leg Shave
(*illustration, top of next page*)

This exercise is probably one that many women do to some extent even if they don't realize it. When shaving your legs, rotate the hips internally (turn the toes in as far as possible)

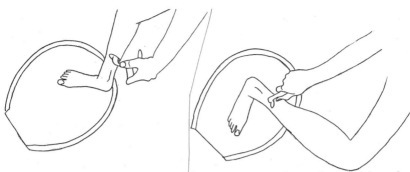

to stretch the hip joint. Then, to get the other side of your leg, rotate your leg externally (turn the foot out as far as it goes). As you rotate the hips as far as you can you should feel a stretch near the hip joint. Try holding this position as you shave.

Exercise #78 - No Handed Rise

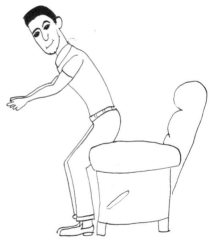

An easy beginning exercise to strengthen lower limb muscles is simply to get out of a chair or off a sofa without using your hands. We often will use our hands to assist us in getting out of a chair or sofa. By not using your hands you make your leg muscles work harder. (This is easier if you scoot to the front of the seat.)

Exercise #79 Hands Up Rise

To add a little degree of difficulty, get out of the

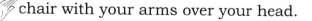
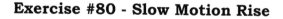

chair with your arms over your head.

Exercise #80 - Slow Motion Rise

This exercise is done to strengthen a number of lower limb muscles that are important for getting in and out of a chair, walking and many sports-specific movements. When getting into or out of a chair (or off the toilet), take 10 to 15 seconds to slowly lower yourself into the seat or conversely slowly raise yourself up into a standing position. This slow muscular contraction will strengthen lower limb muscles to make getting into and out of chairs easier.

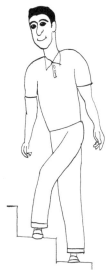

Exercise #81 - Sideways Stair Walk

In order to strengthen some of the hip muscles (especially the hip abductors, which are very important for walking and balancing on one leg at a time) walk up or down any stairs sideways. This motion will work different hip and leg muscles than walking straight ahead.

Exercise #82 - Elevator Button Push

For those of us who often ride in elevators, these two exercises can help you strengthen hip and core muscles and improve your balance. Standing on your stronger leg, stand anywhere from two to four feet away from the buttons, and reach to touch the floor you wish to go to using your opposite foot. You can do this repetitively for a better workout. This exercise is easier to accomplish when there are few, or no, other people in the elevator.

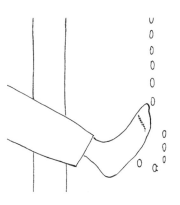

Exercise #83 - Elevator Button Push (Advanced)

Similar to the previous exercise, this one works the hip and core muscles but requires a higher degree of difficulty for balance. While standing on one leg, push the button for the **higher** floor with your foot. This can be quite challenging, especially if you are in a high-rise building.

Exercise #84 - Bathtub/Hamstring Stretch

This is an easy exercise to do in the bathroom when you are getting ready to take a bath. Stand with both feet together about a foot or two away from the bathtub and slowly lean forward at the hips to stretch your hamstrings as you adjust the water temperature. Hold this stretch for 20 to 30 seconds as you turn the knobs or put the plug in the drain.

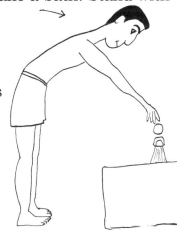

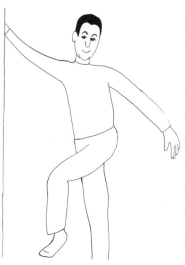

Exercise #85 - Standing Hip Rotator Stretch

This exercise can be done as part of the Door Jamb Series or simply standing anywhere in order to stretch the hip muscles and the lining around the hip (called the capsule) which is prone to getting tight and restricting hip motion. While standing, arms supported for balance if necessary, flex your left hip to where your femur points straight ahead. Your knee can remain bent comfortably. Putting your weight on your right leg, turn your left leg as far to the left as you can while keeping your right foot planted on the ground. You may want to use your hand to gently pull your leg in the same direction for a little more stretch. Repeat with the opposite leg/hip. You should feel a stretch across the back of the hip and buttocks.

Exercise #86 - One Leg Standing Rotations

This exercise works many muscles around the knee and hip including the quadriceps or front thigh muscles. It also works on balance and hip motion. Standing on one leg while doing the dishes, at the bathroom sink or putting on a tie in the morning, turn your body as far as you can to the left and then to the right. This can be done slowly in each direction.

Exercise #87 - TV-SLR or Television Straight Leg Raise

While watching TV or sitting in your favorite chair or on the floor, straighten your leg and raise it up about a foot or two off the ground, hold it for up to 30 seconds and then slowly lower it. This is a good way to get some physical benefit from watching TV. To make it easier to remember, you can do this every time there is a commercial.

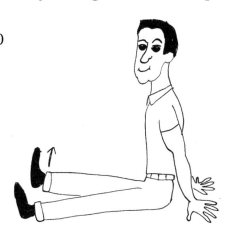

Exercise # 88 - Boring Meeting Quad Set

Sometimes when you want to do something

as simple as exercise #87 but you are in a room with a lot of people and want to get some quadriceps strengthening in, try a simple isometric quadriceps exercise. Simply hold you leg in any specific position, (even with your legs crossed) and tighten your thigh muscles as tight as you can in that specific position. Hold the contraction for 10 to 15 seconds, then relax. Imagine getting some exercise without even moving and not have to totally waste your time in an unwanted meeting.

Exercise #89 - Side Leg Lift

This exercise is similar to exercise #87 but it is done lying on one side or the other. While lying on your right side, lift your right leg about a foot or two. Hold this position for up to 30 seconds and then slowly lower it. Repeat on the other side.

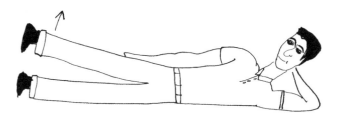

Chapter 9 - Foot and Ankle

The foot and ankle are the bottom of our chain of segments that form our musculoskeletal system. Strength, flexibility, stability and balance are four important elements of proper foot and ankle function. The exercises in this section combine many of these features.

Exercise #90 - Feet Alphabet

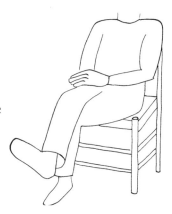

This exercise can be done anywhere you are sitting, except while driving. It should not be hard to find a place. Simply write the alphabet in the air with each of your feet and ankles. You can do the letters in capitals or small letters, and for that matter, in any language you would like. Doing this two or three times on each ankle will begin to strengthen the ankle and maintain or improve motion.

Exercise #91 - Arch Raises

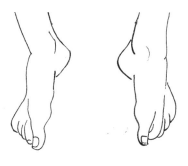

This exercise can be done anywhere you are standing. Simply stand and raise the arch of your foot off the ground (or stand on the outside part of your feet). When you get it up as high as you can, try to hold it for up to 20 seconds, and then slowly lower it down. This can be done one leg at a time, or both together, or when your standing balance is better, even on one foot at time.

Exercise #92 - Sheet Pulls

This is an exercise for first thing in the morning or at night before you go to bed. If you are lucky enough to get a nap every now and then, it may also

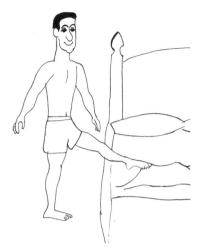

come in handy. Try pulling your sheets up or down using your toes, feet and ankles instead of your hands. It may take a little practice, but you will find that you can use your feet like hands and work some of the small muscles of your feet and ankles.

Exercise #93 - Calf Raises

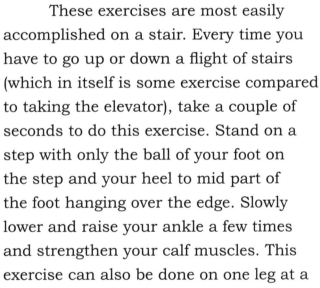

These exercises are most easily accomplished on a stair. Every time you have to go up or down a flight of stairs (which in itself is some exercise compared to taking the elevator), take a couple of seconds to do this exercise. Stand on a step with only the ball of your foot on the step and your heel to mid part of the foot hanging over the edge. Slowly lower and raise your ankle a few times and strengthen your calf muscles. This exercise can also be done on one leg at a time for a more advanced strengthening exercise.

Exercise #94 - Ankle Pumps

This is a simple exercise that anyone can do, anytime, anywhere. It is especially important when you have been sitting in one place for a long time (plane rides, long meetings, commuting in traffic, piano recitals). Simply raise your ankle up (point your toes toward the ceiling) and hold it a few seconds. Then lower in down and point it toward the floor. These exercises help keep the blood circulating in your lower limbs, especially when you have been inactive.

Exercise #95 - Rug Pulls

This exercise can be done in the bathroom if there is a rug on the floor. Alternatively, you can throw a towel on the floor and do the same thing. While sitting on the toilet, grab the towel or rug with your toes and try to curl the rug/towel up just using your toes. This exercise will strengthen the muscles of your feet.

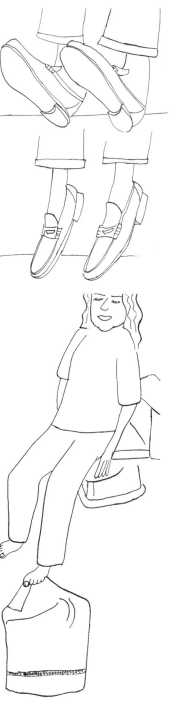

Chapter 10 – Other Balance Exercises

This chapter will describe some other exercises that we have encouraged our patients to try to continue to build hip, pelvic and lower limb strength and balance. Some of these exercises are merely variations on a common theme. They are illustrated here to show you the countless variations you can add to your day-to-day activities to serve as exercises.

Exercise #96 - Goodbye Kiss

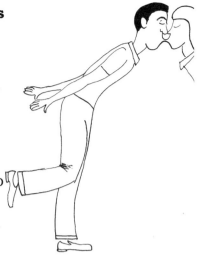

Imagine that! You can get exercise while simply kissing your spouse, children or other loved ones goodbye in the morning (and when you get home in the evening). With the designated person to be kissed sitting or standing close to you, simply lean over to kiss them while standing on one leg. This can be a short duration kiss, where only a little bit of balance and strength is necessary or you may go for the longer, more difficult version, adding romance and love to the increased degree of difficulty from a musculoskeletal perspective. To increase the degree of difficulty (again, from a musculoskeletal perspective, only) try to move further from the desired "kissee."

Exercise #97 - Garbage Drop

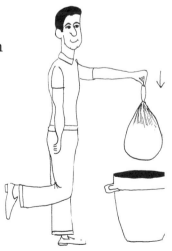

Although not nearly as much fun as exercise #96, this one can be equally effective. When taking the garbage out, stand as far away from the can as possible and slowly lower the garbage in while standing on one leg. This can be very challenging, especially if you have a heavy bag of garbage.

Exercise #98 - Lint or Book Pick Up

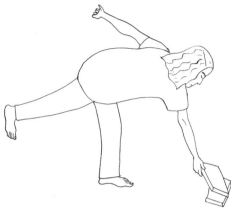

This is still another exercise for standing balance and hip strengthening. It also helps with knee strength. While picking up lint of the floor, or any other of one million things that might be strewn across the floor (this is especially good for teenage kids who may have a lot of work with this exercise), stand on one leg, slowly lower yourself to pick up the object and then slowly return back up to a standing position. This can be done one item at a time until whatever mess on the floor is cleaned up.

Exercise #99 - Laundry Shuffle

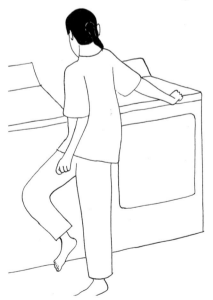

This exercise provides still more fun and excitement while doing a rather boring task like changing the laundry. Stand between the washer and dryer (assuming they are relatively close together or next to each other). Standing on one leg, reach into the washer, grab some clean clothes, pivot on your foot while turning at the hips and maintaining your balance, and then deposit the laundry in the dryer. Trust me, this will make changing the laundry a lot more interesting and musculoskeletally healthy.

Exercise #100 - Doing the Dishes Squat

To add some exercise to doing the dishes, as well as increasing balance, stand on one leg and do partial squats, bending you knee just slightly while washing the dishes. This can be challenging from a strength standpoint (you will feel your quads and gluteal muscles working hard) as well as challenging your standing balance.

Exercise #101 - Red Light Pelvic Floor Squeezes

Pelvic floor exercises strengthen the deep hip and pelvic floor muscles. These muscles can get very weak, particularly in women after they have had children. To strengthen these muscles, squeeze the muscles of yoru lower pelvis like you are holding in your urine because there is no bathroom around. Do this as long as the light is red. Sometimes lightly sucking in your belly button will assist this exercise.

Index of Exercises

Also available from the North American Spine Society

Spine Owner's Manual

A comprehensive guide for patients, the *Spine Owner's Manual* covers anatomy, preventive care, the full spectrum of spinal disorders and degenerative conditions, diagnostic methods and standard treatment options.
Edited by: Marjorie Eskay-Auerbach, MD, JD
110 pp., softcover. ISBN #1-929988-11-7. $9.99

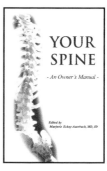

Know Your Spine

This 24-page booklet is a quick guide to spine anatomy and preventive care tips. Give your patients information about exercise, stretching, proper lifting techniques, osteoporosis prevention in this easy-to-read, illustrated format.
24 pp., softcover. ISBN # 1-929988-10-9. $2.99

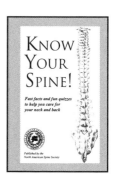

For more information about these books, to find a spine care provider near you, or to learn more about spine health visit the North American Spine Society Web site at www.spine.org, or call toll-free (877) SpineDr.